Dr. Andrew Weil is the leader in the new field of Integrative Medicine, which combines the best ideas and practices of conventional and alternative medicine. A graduate of Harvard Medical School, he is director of the Program in Integrative Medicine at the University of Arizona, the first program to train physicians in this way at an American medical school. He is also the founder of the Center for Integrative Medicine in Tucson, which is advancing the field worldwide. Dr. Weil is well known as an expert in natural medicine, mind-body interactions, and medical botany, as well as the author of the best-selling *Spontaneous Healing* and *8 Weeks to Optimum Health*. According to Dr. Weil, 'Spontaneous healing is not a miracle or a lucky exception, but a fact of biology, the result of the natural healing system that each of us is born with.'

The 'Ask Dr. Weil' program (www.drweil.com) features Andrew Weil, M.D., and is one of the top-rated health sites on the World Wide Web and is featured on Time Warner's Pathfinder Network. The recipient of many awards, it features a daily Q&A with answers to a wide range of health questions, a daily poll, and the Doc Weil Database, which lets readers search hundreds of topics, including material from Dr. Weil's bestselling book *Natural Health, Natural Medicine*. The site also features a Referral Directory (practitioners from acupuncture to Trager work) and DocTalk, a live weekly chat with Dr. Weil. If you have additional questions for Dr. Weil, ask them on his Web site.

By Andrew Weil, M.D.:

Ask Dr. Weil
WOMEN'S HEALTH
YOUR TOP HEALTH CONCERNS
NATURAL REMEDIES
VITAMINS AND MINERALS
COMMON ILLNESSES
HEALTHY LIVING

8 WEEKS TO OPTIMUM HEALTH
SPONTANEOUS HEALING
NATURAL HEALTH, NATURAL MEDICINE
HEALTH AND HEALING
FROM CHOCOLATE TO MORPHINE
THE MARRIAGE OF THE SUN AND THE MOON
THE NATURAL MIND

Ask Dr. Weil

Natural
Remedies

Andrew Weil, M.D.

Edited by Steven Petrow

WARNER BOOKS

A *Warner* Book

First published in Great Britain in 1998 by Warner Books

Published in the United States by Ballantine Books, a division of Random House, Inc., New York 1997

Copyright © Great Bear Productions, LLC 1997

This work was compiled from the *Ask Dr. Weil* Web Site.

The moral right of the author has been asserted.

A CIP catalogue record for this book is available from the British Library

ISBN 0 7515 2608 8

Typeset in Berkeley by M Rules
Printed and bound in Great Britain by Clays Ltd, St Ives plc

Warner Books
A Division of
Little, Brown and Company (UK)
Brettenham House
Lancaster Place
London WC2E 7EN

Introduction

You've taken the first step toward optimum health. This book will give you more information about my philosophy along with answers to some of the questions I am asked most frequently.

I wrote *Spontaneous Healing* and *8 Weeks to Optimum Health* because I wanted to call attention to the innate, intrinsic nature of the healing process. I've always believed that the body can heal itself if you give it a chance. Why? Because it has a healing system. If you're feeling well, it's important to know about this system so that you can enhance your well-being. If you are ill, you'll also want to know about it because it is your best hope of recovery.

To maintain optimum health requires commitment. This book – and the others in the series – can give you much of the basic information you need about diet, supplements, common illnesses, natural remedies, and healthy living.

All of these questions originated on 'Ask Dr. Weil', my program on the World Wide Web. If you still have questions, come visit the clinic at www.drweil.com.

Acupuncture for Fido or Felix?

Q:
Has acupuncture been used to treat cancer in dogs? If not for a cure, at least for pain reduction? Just curious. My beloved dog has inoperable cancer. There doesn't seem to be a lot of literature regarding this.

A:
Acupuncture has been used on animals, including dogs, for arthritis, dysplasia, degenerative nerve conditions, epilepsy, immune system suppression, gastrointestinal problems, and more. In fact, there's an increasing number of holistic veterinarians, and they use acupuncture a lot. This treatment has not been used for cancer in humans, though, and it's never been represented as a cancer treatment. It is, however, very helpful for pain reduction. I think turning to integrative medicine to help your companion is an excellent idea.

Acupuncture works on the principle that life-force energy, called chi (or qi), flows through the body along pathways (meridians) just below the skin's surface. These pathways connect the surface of the body with internal organs and regulate the flow of energy. Acupuncture uses tiny needles to stimulate or fatigue certain points along the meridians and relieve blockage, disperse pain, strengthen muscles and organs, and redirect energy flow.

There are also herbal and nutritional approaches that may help extend life and reduce symptoms in dogs with cancer. I used some of these for my Rhodesian Ridgeback, Coca, when she had bone cancer. I gave her extract of maitake and reishi mushrooms. Maitake, or *Grifola frondosa*, and reishi, *Ganoderma lucidum*, are potent immune boosters. You can find extracts of them in health food stores. I think they helped Coca live much longer and more comfortably than her conventional veterinarian had predicted. She did very well up until the end.

If you decide to see an acupuncturist for your pet, make sure that person has been trained in animal acupuncture. Animal anatomy is different from human.

You may also want to try some acupressure on your own. I'm sure a loving massage by you could do wonders to relieve your dog's pain. *Four Paws, Five Directions*, a book by veterinarian Cheryl Schwartz, offers a comprehensive approach to applying traditional Chinese medicine and acupressure techniques to animals. Try her step-by-step daily massage, which will stimulate your dog's meridians and relax you both.

Beating the Bottle
Naturally?

Q:
What natural herbs have proven effective in battling alcoholism or helpful in curbing the craving for alcohol?

A:
Alcohol can produce true addiction, marked by intense craving, tolerance, and withdrawal. It's a powerful drug, and dependence on it is very resistant to treatment.

A couple of years ago, there was a flurry of excitement over reports that kudzu or ge gen (*Pueraria*) from the south of China was effective as a treatment for alcohol dependence. It's sometimes used as a traditional remedy, and a preparation of the plant was found to reduce cravings for alcohol in strains of hamsters that were bred to be alcoholic. You can find a medicinal preparation of kudzu in Chinese herb stores.

Other than kudzu, I really don't know of any herbal methods for dealing with alcoholism. I'd start by making sure you have good nutrition. In particular, take B vitamins to make up for the B-vitamin deficiency alcoholism can cause. I would suggest one B-100 B-complex a day. Learn other methods of relaxation – like yoga or meditation – to replace alcohol. And get out there and exercise. I would also take two capsules of milk thistle (*Silybum marianum*) twice a day. It protects the liver.

I think the best bet for treating alcoholism is to go to an addiction treatment program. It's really difficult to deal with alcoholism without outside help. For one thing, there's tremendous social pressure to drink – and to drink too much. Consider going to a counseling center or Alcoholics Anonymous, or entering a residential program.

Better Treatments
for Bee Stings?

Q:
A bumblebee and I got into a little rumble the other day and I ended up with a sting in my lower leg. Never did find the sting; but the area around the sting has become quite red and infected. My doc has put me on an antibiotic (cephalexin, 500 milligrams twice a day) for five days. Since I try to use antibiotics only as a last resort, what are the other options for insect stings?

A:
You're wise to avoid overdoing the antibiotics. If your body can beat an infection on its own, it will be more competent to combat future threats. If you override the system with an antibiotic right away, you weaken your own immunity. (There's also the danger of antibiotic resistance. Over time, frequent use of antibiotics leads to the breeding of more virulent bacteria that aren't fazed by existing treatments.)

What to do? Start by using hot compresses on the sting area. The heat dilates the blood vessels and increases healing blood flow to the site of the infection. Also, treat the inflammation locally with full-strength tea tree oil, which is a very effective topical antiseptic. (The oil is extracted from the leaves of *Melaleuca alternifolia*, a tree native to Australia.) Third, do a course of echinacea. Echinacea (*Echinacea purpurea* and related species), familiar to gardeners as purple coneflower, is a natural antibiotic and immune-system enhancer. Try a dropperful of tincture of echinacea in water four times a day for ten days or so. Take at least 1,000 mllligrams of vitamin C twice a day, too.

Only if the infection continues to spread would I then use strong antibiotics. The cephalexin your doctor prescribed would be one choice. It's a semi-synthetic antibacterial, similar to penicillin, originally derived from a microorganism. This is a big gun, so wait a bit and try the other measures first.

As for treatment, for decades the advice concerning the proper way to remove the bee's sting was to scrape it out with something like a blunt knife or a credit card. According to a recent study, you should grab the sting and yank it out as fast as you can. Why the change? According to researchers at the University of California in Riverside, if you pluck out the sting before all the venom is pumped out of it, you'll wind up with a smaller, less painful welt. But you have to act instantaneously to make a difference. The only problem is that while honeybees always leave a sting,

bumblebees rarely do. That's probably why you could-
n't find it. To ease the pain and inflammation, ice the
area immediately and then apply a paste made with
baking soda and water.

Betting or Bailing on Beta-Carotene?

Q:
I've started to take 20,000 IU of beta-carotene a day per your suggestion. Recently I have read that beta-carotene supplements, even in these modest quantities, can be toxic. What is your latest opinion on the subject?

A:
Beta-carotene is not toxic, and there are no studies that suggest it may be. We do have some new information on the supplement, however, that shows it's not the panacea some people had hoped.

The interest in beta-carotene went mainstream after about two dozen studies showed that people with lots of beta-carotene-rich fruits and vegetables in their diets got less cancer and heart disease. As one of the vitamins that neutralize 'free radical' molecules in the body, beta-carotene seemed to make sense as a preventive to oxidative damage leading to cancer.

But the results of giving the vitamin as a supplement were not all encouraging. A Finnish study reported 18 per cent more cases of lung cancer among heavy smokers who took beta-carotene supplements. Then National Cancer Institute researchers halted a study on the effects of beta-carotene and vitamin A. Smokers taking the supplements had 28 per cent more instances of lung cancer than those taking the placebo.

And a twelve-year study of 22,000 physicians found no evidence that beta-carotene supplements were protective against cancer and heart disease.

It's important to note that none of these studies showed that beta-carotene caused cancer. They weren't designed to ask that question. But they do indicate that beta-carotene fails to prevent cancer among smokers. No one is certain why. Some researchers point out that antioxidants can promote free radicals under certain circumstances rather than keeping them under control – and perhaps smoking triggers this action.

It's likely that cancer was already established in the people who were diagnosed with it during these trials. No one believes that antioxidants can cure existing cancers. But study after study has shown the protective effect of high levels of beta-carotene in the blood – and of large amounts of fruits and vegetables in the diet. It is probably not beta-carotene alone that is responsible. It could be the whole family of carotenoid pigments. (And so far, we don't have findings on the effects of beta-carotene in women. The

Women's Antioxidant and Cardiovascular Study is continuing despite the negative findings in men.)

We know of about five hundred carotenoids, the family of substances that the body converts into vitamin A. I recommend taking advantage of them all. Eat a diet rich in fruits and vegetables, especially peaches, melons, mangoes, sweet potatoes, squash, pumpkins, tomatoes, and dark leafy greens. And if you cannot include enough of these in your diet, you may want to take a supplement. I recommend a mixed carotene supplement. Take one capsule (25,000 IU) a day. Enquire in a health food store about these new products.

Does Blue-Green Algae Boost Energy?

Q:
I'm curious about the blue-green algae thing. I was a total disbeliever in the high energy and healing claims many people reported to me, but I was worn down by friends and started taking it. It worked! What do you know and think about this?

A:
Frankly, I don't have any firsthand experience with blue-green algae. Like you, I've heard testimonials from people about its energy-boosting effects. According to what I've read, there is very little research on the chemistry or pharmacology of blue-green algae, but I found one unsettling paper indicating that the species used for commercial purposes is capable of producing liver and nerve toxins, which could be unhealthy in long-term use. Many users report druglike stimulation from these products. Until I know what's responsible for that effect, I'm not going to recommend them. I've seen dozens of sites on the Web and many print advertisements

promoting blue-green algae as a wonder food and an incredible business opportunity. *Caveat emptor*. I'd say wait and see on this. If it works for you, use it, but keep your eye out for new information.

If low energy is a problem for you, you could consider using ginseng, a natural tonic. Used on a regular basis, ginseng increases energy, vitality, sexual vigor, and provides resistance to all kinds of stress. It is nontoxic but Asian ginseng (*Panax ginseng*) can raise blood pressure and is more of a stimulant. I often recommend American ginseng (*Panax quinquefolius*) to people who are chronically ill and to those lacking in vitality.

Vitamin C Aids Recovery from Surgery?

Q:
Have you heard about the intravenous use of vitamin C both before and after surgery to promote faster healing?

A:
Yes. I usually recommend taking 20 grams of vitamin C a day mixed with intravenous fluids, beginning with the IV drip in the operating room and continuing for five days, or until the drip is removed. The problem? Many patients have their requests turned down, either by their doctor or by the hospital pharmacy staff, who are likely to say it's not part of their protocol. Persist. Have your family and friends persist. Say you'll go to another hospital. Then you should be able to get it done. Recently, a friend's brother had surgery for esophageal cancer, and his physician – one of the top gastric surgeons in New York – at first resisted his request for vitamin C, but eventually complied. The result was not surprising to me; the surgeon was so impressed with the speed of healing that he now plans to use vitamin C therapy with other patients.

Care for Some Chicken Soup?

Q:
Is there anything to chicken soup as a cold remedy?

A:
Chicken soup. Just the mention of it conjures up images of steaming broth, packed with carrots, celery, peppercorns, and onion; chunks of chicken; maybe some noodles thrown in. How could it not be a good remedy?

It's comforting, it's warm, and it's fluid. At the University of Nebraska Medical Center, researchers found that chicken soup indeed had anti-inflammatory properties. They discovered that it reduced cold symptoms even when extremely diluted. Apparently the soup inhibits white blood cells called neutrophils, allowing them to fight infection without causing inflammation.

But chicken soup is more than just ingredients. It's comfort, love, and caring, captured in a mixture that fills your nose with fragrant steam and warms your insides. Much of chicken soup's curative power comes from its function as a placebo. (When something has a powerful effect because you believe it will, it's called a placebo.)

Of course, your relationship with chicken soup is affected by your cultural background. In some regions, fish soup is considered the universal elixir. Whatever soup you choose, its benefits also stem from the love and caring it embodies – whether you make the soup yourself or someone gives it to you. It's clear that soup can be a natural remedy that helps you access your own natural healing power.

What's It Take to Lower Cholesterol?

Q:
I have very high cholesterol that is obviously hereditary since I'm a vegetarian and eat no animal products. I consume very little fat, and I take vitamin E. I want to avoid medication. Is there anything I can take in the way of herbs or natural products to lower my cholesterol? And yes, I do exercise regularly.

A:
I'm assuming from your question that you've done all of the standard lifestyle interventions to try to manipulate cholesterol. The primary step, of course, is to reduce saturated fat in your diet as much as possible, meaning mostly fats of animal origin, but also palm and coconut oils. Peanut butter, vegetable oils, shortenings, and margarines can also cause your body to make too much cholesterol. Also cut out coffee, black tea, and cola.

On the positive side, Japanese green tea and foods like onions, garlic, chili peppers, and shiitake mushrooms all have some cholesterol-lowering effects.

Also – as you know – make sure you exercise. (I always recommend thirty minutes, at least five days a week.)

Most people find that changing their eating and exercise habits brings their cholesterol profile down to normal. But everyone's biochemical balance is unique, so these interventions may not have worked for you. If they haven't, then I think it may be time to try niacin, or vitamin B-3.

There have been some ineffective forms of niacin on the market. But there's a new form that definitely works, a wax-impregnated, time-release niacin tablet. J. R. Carlson Laboratories, based in Arlington Heights, Illinois, is one of the companies that make it, in a product called NiacinTime. I would start with a dose of one 500 milligram tablet twice a day with meals.

I will caution you, though, to take niacin with great care and with medical supervision. Time-release niacin is very effective at lowering cholesterol, but it can also disturb liver function. In rare cases, it can cause a toxic fulminant hepatitis. That's a real medical catastrophe that can be fatal.

You must monitor liver function when starting time-release niacin. Have liver function checked at the start of therapy, then test it again after two weeks on niacin. Your doctor will have to arrange the test for you.

As long as your liver enzymes are normal you can stay on the niacin indefinitely, increasing the dose until cholesterol comes down to the level you want. You may want to go up to 1,500 milligrams a day or even higher, but I'll emphasize again that this can only be done with liver monitoring. Keep the dose as low as possible to maintain improvement. You should also know the early signs of liver dysfunction: unexplained loss of appetite, nausea, a feeling of abdominal fullness, abdominal pain, and any other unusual digestive symptoms.

Don't take niacin if you are pregnant or have ulcers, gout, diabetes, gallbladder disease, or liver disease, or have had a recent heart attack.

Niacin seems to both lower the bad LDL (low-density lipoprotein) cholesterol, which damages artery walls, and maybe raise HDL (high-density lipoprotein), the good cholesterol that protects arteries. Your total cholesterol should be under 180. If you can get your total cholesterol under 150, your chance of a heart attack is negligible.

Chromium: Supplement of the Month?

Q:

I've been hearing a lot of talk lately about chromium, both on the news and from some friends in the health business. What exactly does it do, and do you feel it is a beneficial addition to a vitamin diet? Thanks!

A:

You're right, there's a lot of buzz about chromium these days, notably a recent report claiming that chromium produces 'spectacular' results in normalizing glucose and insulin levels in adult-onset diabetes. The U.S. Department of Agriculture study recommended that diabetics take 1,000 micrograms a day.

There's also been a lot of promotion from the manufacturers of one form, chromium picolinate. I often see ads for this product that make unsubstantiated claims like the one opposite.

These are megaclaims: that chromium will help you lose weight, stabilize blood sugar, treat hypoglycemia, lower cholesterol, and improve blood fats.

DIET BOOSTER TABLETS
with Chromium Picolinate

3 STEP FAT ATTACK . . .
Appetite Suppressant to
reduce cravings for food.

Fat Metabolizer for efficient metabolic
breakdown of fats, carbs, and proteins.

Diuretic Action assists in
reducing excess fluids.

CHROMIUM PICOLINATE (200 micrograms)
A natural fat metabolizer. This form
of Chromium plays a vital role in the
functioning of insulin responsible for
regulating the efficient metabolism of
fats, carbohydrates, and protein.

Unless you're diabetic or deficient in chromium – and most people aren't deficient – I don't think supplemental chromium will do anything for you. This is another example of the supplement-of-the-month mentality that we're seeing all the time. We all want to take a pill to solve our problems, and the manufacturers are ready to sell it to us. Enough said.

Charmed by
Colloidal Minerals?

Q:

How do you feel about taking colloidal mineral supplements?

A:

To me these supplements exemplify obnoxious, multi-level marketing in the name of natural medicine. I've received countless copies of an audiotape that advertises colloidal minerals and makes all sorts of unsubstantiated claims. The veterinarian who pitches the stuff is said to have been nominated for the Nobel Prize in medicine. Well, anyone can write a letter to the Nobel Prize committee. I could nominate you for the Nobel Prize in medicine. I have not seen convincing evidence of therapeutic benefit from taking colloidal minerals. And these products may deliver some substances you definitely don't need – aluminum, for example. Well, I feel better after venting.

'Colloidal' means the mineral particles are of a certain size, facilitating use by the body. The marketers will tell you that their products make you live twice as long, protect you from cancer, and cure just about anything. They'll tell you that mineral deficiencies lead to a weakened immune system and cancer. You can buy the products as liquid supplements, aerosols, injectables, and vaginal douches. The literature in health food stores says they're powerful anti-microbials and immune-system stimulants; they're supposed to help cure as many as 650 different diseases. None of these claims is proven.

Some colloidal minerals have a long history as medicinals. In the nineteenth century, for example, colloidal silver was promoted as a treatment for everything from colds to rheumatism. Silver products are useful as germicides, but over time they've been replaced by safer and more effective ones.

There is some potential for harm as well. The body doesn't need silver, and the mineral can accumulate in tissues, causing an irreversible bluish discoloration of the skin. There are even some reports of neurological problems in people who have used oral silver products long-term.

Bottom line: I don't recommend colloidal minerals; there's no reason to think they're as good for you as they are for their marketers. Besides, you should be getting your minerals in highly usable form from fruits and vegetables in your diet. Please eat more fruits and vegetables – organically grown, when possible.

Doubt the
Need to Douche?

Q:

My doctor says this is a growing problem among women: Advertisers try very hard to make women feel unclean so they will buy their products. Douching washes away certain forms of bacteria that protect women from getting infections. When the bacteria aren't there, a woman's body becomes more vulnerable. I'd like to hear your opinion on this.

A:

Douching used to be conventional wisdom, but it's not anymore. Now medical opinion generally discourages women from douching. And when the concern is about hygiene or odor, the risks of douching are much greater than the benefits. Douching can change the pH (or acidity level) of your vagina to be less friendly to helpful bacteria and more attractive to the harmful ones. It can wash away protective flora and leave the tissues more likely to get inflamed or infected.

In her book *Women's Bodies, Women's Wisdom,*

Christiane Northrup, M.D., comments on the way women are taught to believe that the vagina is offensive, requiring deodorants and special sanitization. She says about one-third of all women douche regularly, even though it can cause harm.

There are times, however, that douching can be useful in the short term. For instance, I often recommend douching with acidophilus or diluted tea tree oil for a vaginal infection. You can insert acidophilus culture directly into your vagina in capsule or liquid form. It's a 'friendly' organism that will keep over-aggressive populations of yeast at bay. Tea tree oil is a powerful germicide. Mix about 1½ tablespoons in a cup of warm water to treat yeast infections. Some women are sensitive to this substance; discontinue it at once if you notice any irritation or burning.

Douching also may sometimes serve a protective function. Ejaculation of semen increases the pH of the vagina for eight hours. If you've had intercourse with ejaculation at least three times in a twenty-four-hour period, it will change the pH of the vagina throughout that time and produce conditions more likely for certain bacteria to grow. A douche with 1 tablespoon of white vinegar per pint and a half of warm water will help prevent problems.

Does Echinacea
Fight Colds?

Q:
*Is echinacea helpful in the treatment of colds and flu?
Does it really work as an immune system 'booster' to
help protect against them? What is the proper dosage? Is
it the same for treatment as for prevention? What parts
of the plant should be used?*

A:
Echinacea is a common plant in North America,
cultivated ornamentally in gardens as purple
coneflower. Besides being pretty, it really does work as
an immune system booster. Echinacea is very popular
as a medicinal, and there are hundreds of products
made from it.

There is a great deal of research from Germany show-
ing that echinacea increases the number and activity of
key white blood cells involved in immunity. It is known
to boost the activity of T cells and natural killer cells
and the production of interferon. The herb is versatile
and very safe. Take it at the first sign of a cold or flu –
symptoms like a scratchy throat or achy back.

The root contains the highest concentration of echinacea's active material, although the leaves are also potent. Some products are made from the whole plant; I prefer tinctures made from the root. At the first sign of a cold or flu, take a dropperful of the tincture in a little warm water (or tea) four times a day. Use half that much for children. Make sure the echinacea is potent by putting a bit on your tongue; if it produces a marked numbing sensation after a few minutes, it's good.

I generally don't use echinacea as a preventive, though some people do. The only time I might is if I go on a long plane flight, where the air is recirculated and unhealthy. Then I take echinacea for a couple of days beforehand. To build immunity, you may want to try echinacea at half the adult dosage and stay on it for a while.

There's a popular belief among herbalists that echinacea loses its effectiveness if it's taken continually for more than two or three weeks. But there is no evidence to support that belief, so I think you can go on taking it for as long as you think you need it.

Desperately Seeking Relief from Fleas?

Q:
I'm desperately seeking relief from flea bites and the allergic reaction I get. I have tried numerous internal and external repellents (vitamin B-12, eucalyptus, penny-royal) to no avail. The fleas find me, bite, and cause severe itching over my entire body. This is extremely uncomfortable and upsetting as they are leaving chicken pox-like scarring that lasts for months. Have you any experience with this?

A:
This is a tough one. Fleas love the humid conditions of Hawaii, coastal California, the Gulf Coast, and the Atlantic seaboard south of Maryland. Breeding conditions there are perfect year-round, and with one hundred fleas able to produce a half-million offspring in one month, you can see why they continue to find you.

I'm sorry to say your best hope may be to fumigate your house with chemical 'bombs' available at pet food stores and veterinarians' offices. (Make sure you stay out of your house during the bombing process.) In my experience, the natural repellents that you mention don't work nearly as well as chemical pesticides for severe infestations.

Pyrethrins, active insecticidal agents found in flowers related to chrysanthemums, will kill the fleas and degrade rapidly in the environment. They are nontoxic to humans. You will need to use these or other treatments more than once in order to kill more than one generation of fleas. Growth regulators like the U.S. product fenoxycarb mimic flea hormones and prevent the young larvae from becoming adult fleas.

Another natural product you might try is called Neem but it is not yet available in the U.K. It's a powerful and relatively safe insecticide obtained from a tree in India. You should be able to find it at garden stores. Also, some people dust carpets, furniture, and the crevices where fleas hide out with diatomaceous earth, which contains the fossilized 'skeletons' of sea algae (again, unavailable as yet in the U.K.). Organic farmers often use it to kill insects; its sharp crystals puncture their bodies.

There are biological insecticides that you can try outdoors. Several brands available at lawn and garden stores employ nematodes – tiny worms – that feed on the flea larvae.

You don't say whether you have pets. If you do, try keeping them outside the house. Wash their bedding in hot water and detergent and keep doing so once a week. Also, there's a relatively new product available from vets called Program, which you administer to your pet once a month. Many people have seen dramatic improvement in bad flea situations after starting to use Program.

Once you get things under control, vacuuming every other day may help remove the eggs that fleas lay in the carpet. Get rid of the vacuum bag each time, because the fleas will hatch inside. When you wash the floor, pay special attention to baseboards and areas under the furniture. Shampoo your carpets or bring in a professional steam cleaner at least twice a year. The best way to fight fleas is to keep your environment scrupulously clean.

Forgetting
Something?

Q:
Should I be concerned with forgetting what I was talking about midsentence? It seems like it's getting worse. I'll be saying something and all of a sudden I'll lose my train of thought. Could this be stress? A brain disorder? I am only twenty-seven years old.

A:
Since you're twenty-seven, the cause is probably stress. Stress and anxiety often interfere with memory. Other common causes of memory problems in people in their twenties include smoking marijuana, using other psychoactive drugs like Valium and its relatives, including alcohol.

Memory loss is something to be concerned about. But even with the symptoms you mention, forgetting things is unlikely to be related to a brain disorder in someone your age. I'd like to see what happens if you try some relaxation techniques and eliminate any factors from your life that might be interfering with your memory. The most effective stress reduction technique I know is conscious regulation of breath. For a great breathing exercise see page 63. Regular aerobic exercise and yoga are also good ways to relax and relieve tension.

Another thing to do: Forget about losing your memory. Anxiety about memory can sometimes be a greater problem than actual memory loss, especially in younger people. Americans are particularly susceptible to this. We hear all these public service announcements about Alzheimer's, and they terrify us.

Also, consider how memory works. The secret to memory is attention. If people aren't practised at paying attention, or don't want to pay attention to what's going on, they aren't going to remember. So the problem may be not memory but attention. And the secret to attention is motivation. Unless you're really motivated to pay attention, you may not remember things. And unless you are really motivated and attentive when communicating with the person you're talking to, you may forget what you're saying.

Cure for Hangovers?

Q:
I hate getting out of bed to find myself with quite a splitting reminder of the night before. Is there anything that can help cure the common hangover?

A:
Alcohol is a strong toxin to both the liver and the nervous system, and it irritates the upper digestive tract and urinary system as well. The morning after a binge, you also feel the effects of dehydration. Everyone has a cure for a hangover: sailors claim salt water is the antidote; the Egyptians ate boiled cabbage as a preventive; today, many folks claim it's the 'hair of the dog' that'll stop the hammering. Believe what you will.

I probably don't need to say that moderation is the best way to avoid hangovers. It makes sense to imbibe as much water as possible while you're drinking alcohol, to avoid dehydration. Taking aspirin before drinking, though popular, doesn't help. The best and only surefire remedy is time: as your body metabolizes the toxic overdose, symptoms subside. If you have access to pure oxygen in a canister you can try inhaling some to see if it speeds recovery, but I doubt this is practical for most people. I recommend taking a B-complex vitamin supplement plus extra thiamine (100 milligrams) to counter the B-vitamin depletion caused by alcohol, along with several doses of milk thistle (*Silybum marianum*) to protect the liver. But I really don't know of any hangover treatment that works as well as putting time between yourself and the night before.

Be aware that you should pick your poison wisely. Since alcohol is exempt from most labeling requirements in the U.S.A., it may contain additives that can trigger asthma, migraines, and other reactions. Whenever possible, choose quality brands. The extra money you pour out for a premium cocktail may tax your wallet but will help your liver love you.

Some distilled beverages are rich in substances called congeners, toxic impurities that can greatly add to your woes. Bourbon, rum, and cognac are particularly 'dirty'. Champagne and some sweet wines are also notorious causers of hangovers. Vodka, being just pure alcohol and water, is the cleanest.

It's always a good idea to pace yourself, and to eat if you have more than a drink or two.

My drink of choice is sake, which seems pretty clean to me. I don't get a hangover from it, even when I drink more than normal. *Kanpai!*

Natural Remedies
for Hay Fever?

Q:
During the spring and summer I suffer from minor hay fever (sneezing, irritated and swollen sinuses). For years I've kept it under control with over-the-counter drugs like Sudafed. I'd like to stop taking these drugs. Are there any natural remedies?

A:
As you've found, conventional treatments for hay fever aren't very good. Desensitization shots are expensive, can hurt, and are risky. Antihistamines often reduce itching, dry up a runny nose, and quiet down a sneezing attack, but because they act on the brain, they can make you drowsy and depressed. Recently, new antihistamines have been developed that aren't absorbed into the brain (Clarityn, for example). They may have different side effects, they don't work for everyone, and they're not cheap Steroid drugs are even stronger than antihistamines. Doctors often prescribe steroid nasal inhalers (like Beconase) for hay fever. They can be very effective,

but the steroids are bound to get into your system, and these hormones weaken our immune systems.

My objection to all these drugs is that they suppress or block the allergic process and, in doing so, only perpetuate the disease by frustrating it. I've had intense ragweed allergy all my life and I know that it's possible to make things better by changing your lifestyle and attitude.

Stinging nettle (*Urtica dioica*) is the best natural remedy that I know. It's most effective taken in a freeze-dried form sold as a capsule. The dose is one to two capsules every two to four hours as needed. Stinging nettle is completely nontoxic and spectacularly effective in controlling hay fever symptoms.

Can I Take an
Herbal Overdose?

Q:

I would like to know whether there is any herb that one could consume to excess and therefore suffer health problems. I consume 25 grams of raw ginger, 25 grams of raw garlic, and 20 grams of eleuthero, or Siberian ginseng (Eleutherococcus senticosus) every day. Are there any dangers in doing so? I also plan to take triphala, ashwagandha, barley green, sun chlorella, echinacea, Ginkgo biloba, and gotu kola. Is there any harm in taking any of these products in the same or larger quantities?

A:

That's a lot of herbs to take every day, and I have to wonder what health problems you're using them for. In general, I think it's a shame to waste medicinal herbs by taking them just because they're there. They'll work better for you if you save them for the times when your body needs special attention.

I think any herb can be taken in excess. For example, there have been a few reported cases of bleeding problems in people taking very large amounts of garlic, which can act as an anticoagulant. Some herbalists also say that too much garlic can deplete your intestinal flora and make it harder to absorb nutrients.

I think the amounts of ginger and garlic you're talking about are fine. But I wonder about swallowing a whole grab bag of herbs, unless you're taking them for specific reasons.

Herbs are dilute forms of natural drugs, not health foods or dietary supplements. You shouldn't take them casually or for no reason, any more than you would take pharmaceutical drugs casually or for no reason. Any herb that produces a therapeutic effect can also cause side effects. And, just as for any drug, it's important to watch for sensitivities particular to your body.

Unless you have specific illnesses you are treating, I'd back off from the herbal cornucopia. If you use herbs just because you think it's healthy to do so, you may build up a resistance to their effects. Then you won't have them available to work for you if you get sick and really need them.

Need a Quickie
for a Hickey?

Q:
What's the best way to get rid of a hickey?

A:
First of all, there's no quick fix for a hickey or lovebite. It's just a plain old bruise, and basically you wait for it to heal. My advice is to tell your partner either not to kiss so hard next time or not to kiss so high above your collar line. You could try ice right away on the injured area, but that might interrupt the heat of the moment. (A friend of mine puts a tablespoon in his freezer and then applies the cold spoon to the hickey for the same effect.) Fortunately, hickeys aren't life-threatening or permanently disfiguring; like any bruise, they'll begin to fade in a few days. If you're shy about walking around with a red splotch on your neck, try my favorite remedy: a poloneck shirt.

You can experiment with a few things while you wait it out. Rub in a little tincture of arnica or arnica gel. Arnica comes from a plant in the daisy family that grows in the Rocky Mountains, and it's wonderful for bruises, sprains, and sore muscles. Aloe vera, from a succulent plant native to Africa, also soothes skin irritation. Kathi Keville, author of *Herbs for Health and Healing*, makes a bruise compress with the following:

1 tablespoon tincture of arnica
a smidgen of Saint-John's-wort flowering tops
a smidgen of witch hazel bark or chamomile flowers
4 drops lavender essential oil
2 tablespoons cold water

Soak a flannel in the liquid, wring it out, and place it directly on your hickey.

Kombucha Tea
for HIV?

Q:
I'm infected with HIV and am wondering what you think about the Kombucha mushroom for someone with a weakened immune system. I've been drinking the tea for two months and so far consider the effects nothing short of miraculous.

A:
First, the Kombucha mushroom is not a mushroom. It's a mixed culture of several species of bacteria and yeasts that is reported to have immune-boosting and antibiotic properties. Kombucha has become popular because of some initial positive press about its beneficial effects and because it's readily available.

If you're getting good effects, go ahead and use it. But generally I'm cautious about recommending it for two reasons. The first is that the culture can become contaminated with dangerous organisms; this would be of special concern for anyone whose immune system was suppressed. There are reports of a number of serious reactions, including deaths, among users of

Kombucha mushrooms apparently due to contamination. If the culture develops an unusual odor or color, throw it out. Second, I'm not enthusiastic about people taking antibiotics of any kind without good reason.

I've heard a few dramatic stories of improvement among people with HIV and reports of higher energy levels and mental acuity. But we really have no research on Kombucha. All of the reports, like yours, are testimonials. People with HIV who have low T cell counts should be sure to talk to their physician before taking Kombucha.

In general the people with HIV who have done well are those who are using the protease 'cocktail' (a powerful combination of anti-HIV drugs) and who have worked to improve their total lifestyle – diet, stress reduction, exercise, sexuality, and emotional life.

How to Avoid
the Nit Picking?

Q:

Any thoughts on treatment of head lice? We had a persistent case last year. Our pediatrician recommended Rid. I followed the directions to the letter, but the lice seem to be resistant. Only manual removal of lice and nits worked. If this happens again, do you know of an easier method?

A:

These tiny flat parasites are about the size of a sesame seed, and move from person to person by way of combs, hats, and personal contact. If you have kids in school, this might become a problem in your household. If you take a close look at the child's scalp with a magnifying glass, you can see little grayish-white eggs, or nits, attached to the hair shafts. You rarely see the adult lice.

U.S. preparations like Rid and Kwell work to kill lice, but they are definitely toxic to people, too. The conventional treatment is 1 per cent lindane (sold as Kwell in the U.S.A.) in a shampoo, cream, or lotion applied once a day for two days (lindane is no longer used in products in the U.K.) Then you can comb the eggs out of the hair, row by row, using a fine-tooth comb. Lotions made with 0.5 per cent malathion such as Prioderm can also work. But both of these can be irritating and are flammable. Lindane is a cousin of DDT, and can harm the nervous system.

Organisms resistant to these treatments are increasing, and recurrence is common. It may be that you were seeing reinfection, or that enough of the eggs survived to make a comeback. Sometimes it's necessary to go back at the nits after they hatch (in about ten days). Also, you have to get rid of or properly clean all sources of the lice: combs, hats, clothing, rugs, even chair coverings (cleaning includes vacuuming, laundering, steam pressing, or dry cleaning).

For a safe treatment, I would consider Neem. Neem, derived from a tree in India, is sold in garden shops as a pesticide. You'll find it in stores that carry organic gardening supplies.

Another treatment people have found helpful is an herbal recipe consisting of 2 ounces of vegetable oil, 20 drops of tea tree oil, and 10 drops each of the following essential oils: rosemary, lavender, and lemon. Do a skin test on the inside of the elbow first, and wait several hours to make sure the strong oils don't irritate the skin. Leave the mixture on the infected head under a towel for an hour, then shampoo. You'll probably have to repeat this at least once to get rid of the next batch of hatched lice.

If you use any of these treatments, make sure your child's eyes are covered and that you apply the pesticide only to the head and neck.

Lice are awful for children because the itching is so severe. The easiest way to deal with these insects is to avoid getting them, if at all possible (and sometimes that's difficult). Make sure your children don't share pillows, hats, combs, or hairbrushes with others. If there's an infestation at school, change the bedsheets often. Wash them in hot water and dry them in the dryer. Wash combs and brushes, and soak them in hot water for ten minutes. Check your children for head lice at least once a week, looking for nits behind the ears and above the neck.

Lice have made a major comeback in schools these days, so you have to stay on the lookout.

Better Methods for Treating Lupus?

Q:

Are there any homeopathic medicines that are good for treating lupus?

A:

Lupus is a serious autoimmune disease that is imperfectly managed by conventional medicine. It can be mild or life-threatening and may cause a variety of symptoms, including arthritis, skin eruptions, neurological problems, and kidney disease. Four times as many women as men have lupus, and there isn't much known about its cause. Some think a viral infection may trigger the immune-system dysfunction.

The drugs that conventional doctors use for lupus are immune-suppressive and toxic. They may be necessary when symptoms are most severe, but they reduce the chance that the disease will go into remission naturally.

Homeopathic medicine would not be my first choice to treat lupus. Instead, I've seen very good results in patients who modify their diet and use anti-inflammatory supplements and herbs like black currant oil, ginger, turmeric, and feverfew, in addition to mind-body healing techniques, like hypnotherapy and guided imagery.

You may also want to experiment with Native American, Ayurvedic, or Chinese medicine. I'd start by eating as little protein as possible and eliminating dairy products. Try to get lots of starches and fresh fruits and vegetables.

Eat sardines packed in sardine oil (without salt) three times a week, or take supplemental linseed meal. These provide omega-3 fatty acids. Black currant oil is a natural source of another fatty acid called gamma linolenic acid (GLA), which is an effective anti-inflammatory. Take 500 milligrams twice a day. Take feverfew (*Tanacetum parthenium*), an anti-inflammatory herb, to help with any arthritis (one capsule of the freeze-dried leaves twice a day for as long as you notice symptoms).

Exercise regularly. If you're hurting from arthritis, swimming can bring relief. Drink plenty of water and get lots of rest. Seek out ways to avoid stress and fatigue in your life.

It's especially important not to stay with a conventional doctor who encourages you to feel hopeless or negative. Lupus has a high potential to go naturally into remission, and the attitude of your physician can powerfully influence your ability to feel well. For insight into one woman's encounters with conventional and alternative medicine in her efforts to manage this disease, read Laura Chester's book *Lupus Novice: Towards Self Healing*.

Healing
with Magnets?

Q:
A member of my family has consulted a healer regarding her general health, and was given magnets in order to correct her magnetic field. She is to place the left foot on one magnet and the right foot on a different magnet every day. The healer told her that this will correct imbalances caused by strong electromagnetic fields such as the ones in New York's subway system. Is this use of magnets safe, and can it be beneficial?

A:
Magnet therapy is growing in popularity after a long history rooted in the ancient cultures of China, India, and Egypt. There are various theories on the effects of magnets on the body and all sorts of claims as to their power. Roger Coghill, a British scientist, theorizes that magnets affect the iron in red blood cells, improving the blood's oxygen-carrying ability. Others say magnets stimulate nerve endings and modify electrical processes in the body. They suggest that magnets can help counteract electro-magnetic

pollution from devices like microwave ovens and television sets (and the New York subway system, I suppose). Frankly, we don't know a lot about the positive or negative medical effects of magnets and magnetic fields. Researchers are just beginning to explore this area.

People use magnets to relieve pain, accelerate healing, and boost mental and physical energy. For example, to relieve a toothache, magnet devotees will place the north magnetic pole of a magnet against the cheek for fifteen to twenty minutes. Putting the north pole on the forehead between your eyebrows for ten minutes at bedtime is supposed to lead to better sleep after a few days.

A number of Japanese magnetic devices are available for relief of pain, such as the pain of arthritis. You can buy magnet insoles, magnet mattress pads, magnet carseat covers, and small magnets to place on various parts of your body. I've met patients who swear by them, but I don't think we can assume that wearing magnets is necessarily healthful – or helpful. Also, these devices are quite expensive.

Some people say that while contact with a south magnetic pole is relaxing, contact with a north magnetic pole can be stimulating and might activate latent tumors or other disease processes. Until the new field of energy medicine really gets going, I think we'll have to experiment on our own and watch for results of studies as they appear. For an overview of the subject written by an enthusiast, look up *Discovery of Magnetic Health: A Health Care Alternative* by George J. Washnis and Richard Z. Hricak.

Do Mosquitoes
Love You?

Q:

Are there any natural ways to prevent getting mosquito bites? Once you've been unlucky enough to get bitten, are there any ways to stop the itch and swelling?

A:

Mosquitoes are definitely attracted to some people more than others. And some people react more strongly to mosquito bites than others. I'm no fan of chemical sprays like Off! because the active ingredient – Deet – feels nasty and is toxic.

You can try using one of the natural insect repellents that you'll find in health food stores. Frankly, though, I think these work only if the mosquitoes are not too populous, and if you apply the stuff very frequently.

Some friends swear by Skin-So-Soft, a bath oil made by Avon, which seems to offer some protection. Other ways to escape include going indoors at mosquito feeding time – usually at dusk – or wearing long-sleeve, loose-fitting clothing and tucking your trousers into your socks. Black and white fabrics seem to attract the insects. So all you downtown types might go for earth tones when in the country.

Once you're bitten, you can try a couple of things. I use a bit of red Tiger Balm dabbed on the bite to distract myself from the itching. Some people use aloe vera.

If you can reduce your allergic responsiveness through changes in your diet or mental attitude, mosquito bites may not bother you so much. Try eating garlic or reducing the protein in your diet. (High levels of protein can irritate the immune system, aggravating your reactivity.)

You may also want to try taking B-complex vitamins regularly during the summer months. Mosquitoes seem to find some people's blood a little less palatable after a few weeks of the supplements.

Bothered by
a Nosebleed?

Q:
*Any cure for nose-bleeding? What is the scientific name
for it?*

A:
Nosebleeds can look fairly dramatic because of all
that bright red blood running down your face. But
they're actually more of a bother than a medical problem – and definitely not life-threatening. Sometimes a
nosebleed can be a symptom of something else, such
as high blood pressure or a clotting disorder. But most
often it's spontaneous and more likely to happen in
winter than in any other season. When the lining of
your nose dries out or there's a lot of sneezing or
nose-blowing because you have allergies or a cold,
the blood vessels close to the surface can rupture.
This may happen when you're spending a lot of time
in overheated rooms, or it may happen when someone punches you in the nose.

The first thing to do if you get a nosebleed is to

blow your nose gently. Don't lean back. Instead, sit upright or lean your head slightly forward and pinch both nostrils. Hold them shut for five to ten minutes and breathe through your mouth. By plugging your nose, you stop the blood flow and allow the blood vessels to form a clot. If the bleeding hasn't stopped after ten minutes, spray some decongestant into your nose. This shrinks the blood vessels and aids in repair. Then hold your nose again for ten minutes.

Another way to stop bleeding is to sniff a little bit of powdered yarrow. Yarrow, or *Achillea millefolium*, has a wonderful ability to stop bleeding.

If after twenty minutes you're still bleeding, it's best to go to a doctor to get the blood vessels sealed off with some silver nitrate solution. You'll also likely need professional help if you're taking blood thinners or large doses of aspirin.

Once you've stopped bleeding, don't blow your nose for a while or exert yourself – the bleeding could start up again.

If you live in a dry climate, one solution to regular nosebleeds is to use a humidifier in your home. Another option is to rub some liquid vitamin E in your nose. You can also try taking vitamin C as a supplement – at least 1,000 milligrams twice a day – since it decreases the fragility of small blood vessels. Another possibility is bilberry extract (from the

European blueberry, *Vaccinium myrtillus*), which does the same thing.

By the way, the scientific name for nosebleed is 'epistaxis'.

SOS for PMS?

Q:

I am a victim of premenstrual syndrome (PMS). It has become progressively worse in the past year, I'd say. My moods are so extreme, it is difficult for me to be around other humans. I go from being filled with rage and hostility to feeling anxious and scared for no reason, to sobbing uncontrollably at the drop of a hat. I recently went on the Pill, which has made my cycle more predictable, but I'm still an emotional basket case. My boyfriend is ready to kill me. Please help.

A:

Many male doctors consider PMS an imaginary condition, and some feminists believe it's a construct of the male establishment. Nevertheless, many women suffer severe physical discomfort, plus the mood swings you mention, just before the onset of menstruation. Common symptoms include depression, tension, anger, difficulty concentrating, lethargy, changes in appetite, and a feeling of being overwhelmed. These can be accompanied by breast tenderness, headache, fluid retention, and joint or muscle pain. PMS's effects may begin around the time of ovulation, then diminish during menstruation or just after.

It is possible to ease the severity of PMS or even eliminate it entirely. First, I'd suggest removing all caffeine – including chocolate – from your life. Many women crave chocolate just before menstruation and say it acts as an antidepressant. But it can be addictive and can have a powerful effect on moods, energy cycles, and sleep patterns. Caffeine adds to nervous tension and increases your heart rate. (So beware of using caffeine or chocolate as a spiritual or emotional salve.) Also avoid all polyunsaturated vegetable oils, which can promote inflammation.

Next, you should exercise regularly. I would suggest thirty minutes of some sustained aerobic activity five days a week. Besides giving a sense of strength and well-being, and increasing the flow of oxygen to all organs, exercise helps to regulate your hormone levels.

Third, take a supplement of evening primrose oil or black currant oil, two capsules two or three times a day. Both supplements supply an unusual fatty acid called gamma-linolenic acid (GLA), an effective anti-inflammatory agent. (GLA also promotes healthy skin, hair, and nails.) Try this for at least two months and continue if you feel better. I also would take supplements of calcium and magnesium, preferably

1,200 to 1,500 milligrams of calcium citrate at bedtime, and half that amount of magnesium. These may ease menstrual cramps.

You might experiment with several herbs that have a good track record with PMS. The first is dong quai, a Chinese remedy made from the root of *Angelica sinensis*, in the carrot family. It acts as a general tonic for the female reproductive system in much the same way that ginseng works for men. You can try two capsules twice a day for several months to see how it affects you. Another possibility is vitex, or chaste tree (*Vitex agnus-castus*), in the same dosage. It helps regulate the female reproductive cycle. Try these one at a time to assess their benefit.

As a general tonic for your mind, body, and moods, experiment with deep breathing and other relaxation techniques. It may also be helpful to analyze which symptoms you are feeling and when. Try listing the symptoms that bother you most, then recording when you experience them during the month. This can help you be aware of what to expect each month, and also clarify which symptoms are actually tied to your menstrual cycle and which might have another cause.

Is Rolfing Better
than Massage?

Q:
I'd like to know your opinions on Rolfing and if you think it is a more beneficial form of massage than others. Thanks.

A:
Rolfing is not simply massage. It's a form of body work intended to restructure the connective tissue, or fascia. Basic Rolfing consists of ten intensive sessions in which the practitioner applies firm – even painful – pressure with the fingers and elbows to specific parts of the body. For people who are open to Rolfing, it can be a great way to get more in touch with your body and change long-standing problems of bad posture and chronic pain (like back pain). Rolfing can also release repressed emotions as well as diminish habitual muscle tension. If you want to make some kind of change in your life and work on your body, you might consider Rolfing. For a referral in your area, write or call the Institute of Complementary Medicine (see Other Resources, page 82).

Commit to
Quit Smoking?

Q:
I know I should quit. I just can't seem to. I desperately need help.

A:
I know that many smokers stare at themselves in the mirror, asking, 'How do I quit?' It's hard. Tobacco in the form of cigarettes is the most addictive drug in the world – right up there with crack cocaine. There are two reasons for this: Nicotine is one of the strongest stimulants known, and smoking is one of the most efflcient drug-delivery systems. Smoking actually puts drugs into the brain more directly than intravenous injection.

In the early part of this century, cigarette smoking was accepted, and was even considered healthful and glamorous. It was thought to promote mental acuity, efficiency, and relaxation. It is true that one of the 'benefits' of smoking is a brief relief of internal tension; unfortunately, within twenty minutes the tension is back, stronger than before, and the brain demands another fix.

Low-tar, low-nicotine cigarettes offer no great advantages. People tend to smoke more of them, or inhale more deeply to get the same amount of nicotine. Pipes and cigars, if the smoke is not inhaled, do not cause lung cancer and emphysema, but they do increase the risk of oral cancer (as do snuff and chewing tobacco).

I feel so strongly about the health risks of smoking that I will not accept patients who are users unless they are willing to try to quit. Many programs can help you: acupuncture, hypnotherapy, and support groups. There are also a slew of new devices on the market – nicotine patches and gum, for instance – that work for some. None of these methods works reliably for everyone. Most successful quitters do it on their own after one or more unsuccessful attempts. Going 'cold turkey' also seems to work better than gradually cutting down.

Don't get discouraged. If you can't quit today, you may be able to tomorrow. Motivation is the key, and it can come only from you. Remember: You get credit for every attempt you make. In fact, the best predictor for success is making attempts to quit.

If you smoke, do this breathing exercise. It will help motivate you to quit and help you with your cravings for cigarettes when you do. Here's how:

1. Sit with your back straight. Place the tip of your tongue against the ridge of tissue behind your upper front teeth and keep it there throughout the exercise.
2. Exhale completely through your mouth, making a *whoosh* sound.
3. Close your mouth and inhale quietly through your nose to a mental count of four.
4. Hold your breath for a count of seven.
5. Exhale completely through your mouth, again making a *whoosh* sound, to a count of eight.
6. This is one breath. Now inhale again and repeat the cycle three more times.

Do this throughout the day, whenever you crave a smoke.

If you smoke, you should take antioxidant vitamins and minerals, which to some extent can reverse the changes in respiratory tissue caused by tobacco, and so help protect against lung cancer. Also, increase your intake of dietary sources of carotenes (carrots, sweet potatoes, yellow and orange squash and fruits, and leafy green vegetables).

Good luck, and please set a date for your next attempt to quit.

Cut Out
That Snore?

Q:
Outside of a drastic operation, what can I do to reduce or eliminate snoring?

A:
Snoring results when the soft tissue of the airway relaxes and vibrates during sleep (this also may happen when your nose is obstructed while you try to breathe). It can range in severity from a bothersome nuisance to real difficulty getting oxygen during the night. So far, the loudest recorded snore has been 88 decibels, potentially enough to cause hearing loss with prolonged exposure. Snoring is three times more common in obese people, and its frequency increases with age. I've seen a variety of estimates, but many agree that about 60 per cent of men and 40 per cent of women snore. Snoring tends to occur more often when people sleep on their backs, because of the position of the airway structures.

There are several devices that are claimed to help snorers. One product in the U.S.A. is a battery-operated wristband called the Mini Snore Control that's activated by sound. When you start snoring, the device begins to vibrate and wakes you enough so you can roll over on your side. Usually that's enough to stop the snore.

Another device fits on the nose and keeps the nasal passages open. It looks fairly easy to use and the manufacturer claims it dramatically reduces snoring. There are also pillows that keep the head and neck in a better position to avoid snoring. But I'm less enthusiastic about those.

What else can you do? Avoid alcoholic beverages, tranquilizers, sleeping pills, or antihistamines before going to bed. Try to sleep on your side or your stomach. Also, consider the possibility that you may have a nasal infection or allergy that is clogging your nose.

There is an operation to end snoring, as you say. Surgeons cut the uvula, the little organ that hangs down in the back of the throat, and get success in two-thirds of cases. But this surgery is painful and should only be used as a last resort.

I also recommend telling your sleeping partner that it's fine for him or her to wake you, roll you, or do whatever's necessary – other than asphyxiate you – to get you to stop. Pleasant dreams.

Cramped by Stitches?

Q:
*When running, I get what often is referred to as a stitch —
a pain in the abdominal area just below the rib cage.
What causes this? What can I do for it?*

A:
The pain you're feeling is probably a spasm of one of
the muscles in the abdominal wall or between the
ribs. The cause could be any one of many possi-
bilities. Perhaps you're running in a way that puts an
unequal strain on a particular muscle. You may be
more fatigued than you realize. Or you may be
depleted in sodium or potassium from exertion.
Cramps like this aren't very well understood, but it's
believed they involve depletion of muscle nutrients,
fluid loss, and electrolyte imbalance.

Stretching more before running probably won't
make any difference. Even the best-conditioned ath-
letes get stitches unpredictably. Interestingly (and
ironically), people who do not exercise regularly and
are in poor condition are less likely to get them.

I'll admit stitches can really hurt, but I don't think

the abdominal pain you're experiencing is anything to be concerned about. It can be so strong, though, that you lose your balance and fall. Maybe it's just a sign that you should stop your run right then and rest a little bit.

To ease the pain, gently stretch the muscle. If you've made it home and you still hurt, apply an ice pack to relax the muscle and reduce swelling.

If you want to provide your muscles with more energy, herbs can help your body process carbohydrates and absorb oxygen more efficiently. They also can boost muscle recovery after exercise. You can try licorice, ginseng, or schizandra berries to boost your muscles' stamina. Kathi Keville offers a recipe incorporating all of them in *Herbs for Health and Healing*:

1 teaspoon tincture of Siberian ginseng root
½ teaspoon each tinctures of shizandra berries, ginseng root, saw palmetto berries, and licorice root

Combine ingredients. Take ½ dropperful twice a day, or as needed for stamina.

Does Transcendental Meditation Work?

Q:

Transcendental meditation (TM) proponents maintain that the technique has far-reaching stress-reduction benefits, even going as far as to say it 'can reverse the signs of aging' if practiced correctly. Are you familiar with any medical studies that have attempted to confirm the claims of TM enthusiasts?

A:

Transcendental meditation (TM) first became popular in the United States in the 1960s when the Beatles, Mia Farrow, the Beach Boys, and other celebrities took it up. The practice, based on ancient yogic teachings, applies a simple meditation technique that involves the repetition of a Sanskrit word or phrase – called a mantra – to prevent distracting thoughts. The four key elements to eliciting a relaxation response are a quiet environment, an object to dwell upon (like a word or symbol), a comfortable position, and, most important, a passive attitude that allows thoughts, images, and feelings to drift into your awareness and pass on through. Meditation is a way to break addiction to thought – to place your attention in present reality.

Proponents of TM have made some extreme claims that their method will reverse the effects of aging, allow people to levitate, and cause them to reach enlightenment. I'm sorry to say I haven't seen evidence for any of this, and you're wise to question them. But here's the good news. Studies on TM at Harvard Medical School in the mid-seventies showed it to lower oxygen consumption, increase blood flow, and slow heart rate, leading to a deep relaxation. Researchers also found TM to lower levels of blood lactate, which is associated with anxiety, and to decrease blood pressure in people with hypertension. You might look at Herbert Benson's book *The Relaxation Response*, which offers an excellent overview of this research.

I believe that other forms of meditation offer similar benefits, and, unlike TM, many are free. I don't recommend meditation for everyone; some people aren't ready for it, and some need simpler techniques for relaxing.

Help for
Tummy Trouble?

Q:
*People like me with stomach complaints such as heart-
burn, abdominal bloating, or gas pains are generously
prescribed drugs such as Pepcid, Zantac or Tagamet.
Most of these drugs have potential long-term side effects,
usually underplayed by Western doctors. Could you recommend gentler, natural remedies for these problems?
Also, what lifestyle changes may help?*

A:
Digestive disorders often can be traced to poor eating
habits and stress. The gastrointestinal tract is very
susceptible to the disturbing influence of stress,
because it relies on complex coordination by the
autonomic nervous system.

The licorice extract DGL (deglycyrrhizinated
licorice) is an excellent natural remedy for all the
problems you mention. DGL increases the mucous
coating of the stomach, making it more resistant to
the effects of acid. It is nontoxic and inexpensive, and
it works better than prescription drugs. The

prescription drugs act by suppressing acid production in the stomach. The problem with this approach is that you're not really getting to the root problem. As soon as you stop taking these drugs, there's going to be a rebound production of acid. If you deal with the problem by using DGL, you increase the body's defensive strength.

DGL is available as tablets or powder. Chew one to two tablets or take ¼ teaspoon of the powder fifteen minutes before meals and again at bedtime. Allow the material to dissolve slowly in your mouth and run down your throat.

For stomach problems generally, a number of herbal remedies can help. Peppermint tea is wonderful for nausea, indigestion, and some cases of heartburn (but because it relaxes the sphincter where the esophagus joins the stomach, it can worsen esophageal reflux syndrome, in which stomach acid irritates the lower esophagus). In general, it soothes the lining of the digestive tract. Buy pure peppermint tea, brew it in a covered container to retain the volatile components, and drink it hot or iced. Chamomile is also excellent for heartburn and indigestion, and will not aggravate esophageal reflux. You can buy it in tea bags in the supermarket. Steep in hot water in a covered container for ten minutes, and then enjoy.

I also feel strongly that people with stomach

problems should not rely solely on remedies. Try looking for the causes of your problems, which probably have to do with excess consumption of stomach irritants like coffee, other forms of caffeine, decaffeinated coffee, alcohol, and foods (or food combinations) that you don't tolerate well. Smoking is another cause of stomach distress. I'd encourage you to make some dietary experiments to see if you can reduce symptoms and thereby eliminate the problem. A simple rule: Pay attention to – and stop eating – what makes your stomach hurt. Try eating smaller amounts more frequently. And work on reducing stress in your life.

Is Urine the
Water of Life?

Q:

Not long ago, Yoga Journal *had an article on urine therapy. This is quite a bugaboo for those of us in the West. The article referred to a book,* Your Own Perfect Medicine, *which really sang the praises of pee! Do you have any experience with this treatment, and if so, what is your opinion of it?*

A:

Urine therapy refers to the drinking of one's own urine for therapeutic benefit. This unusual practice originated in India. Occasionally, I come across folk remedies in our culture involving topical applications of urine, which I have no problem with. Enough people report good effects with it in conditions like athlete's foot and jellyfish stings to make me think it works, and I am not upset at the thought of having urine on the skin.

But the drinking of urine is a different matter. Some proponents of urine therapy say you can rid yourself of herpes, AIDS, and leprosy by drinking your own urine. Not long ago, about 600 proponents gathered in India for three days to compare notes on the practice, which they claimed could reverse conditions ranging from arthritis to cancer. Those who recommend urine therapy point to the complexity of the fluid and relate its components to the life-giving properties of blood.

When I think about drinking urine, I find myself up against a major psychological barrier. There are two parts to this: a gut-level revulsion and an intellectual conviction that urine drinking violates a clear intent of the body to rid itself of waste. As a practitioner of natural medicine, I find it hard to get past the idea that the body wants to get rid of urine. Urine does contain hormones and other bioactive substances that might produce therapeutic effects. But my impression is that the benefits being reported are placebo responses activated by confronting and breaking a powerful psychological taboo. I would not stand in the way of anyone who wanted to try urine therapy, but for myself and my family, I prefer to seek out treatments that are more to my taste.

How to Beat
the Winter Blues?

Q:
What have you heard about SAD (seasonal affective disorder)? Since I was diagnosed, I have been experimenting, and a few years ago reasoned that if feverfew affects serotonin uptake for migraines, it might work for SAD. It has been quite beneficial used in conjunction with full-spectrum lighting.

A:
Winter is the time of year when people with seasonal affective disorder start to feel bad. People who have it usually know it – but not always. It's a depression, often severe, that comes on in winter months and is believed to be related to lack of exposure to light. People feel lethargic, irritable, and depressed; many crave carbohydrates and tend to gain weight. It's more common in the northern latitudes, affecting many people in Alaska, for example, and few here in southern Arizona. Twice as many women as men experience this disorder.

There are two treatments recommended for SAD.

First, exposure to a small amount of full-spectrum light has really helped some people. Even ordinary artificial light seems to work – at least thirty minutes a day at 10,000 lux (20 times normal indoor lighting). It may take three to four weeks to feel the full effect. It would also be a good idea to exercise outdoors in the middle of the day, looking up toward the sky (but not directly into the sun) now and then. The authority on light treatment for SAD is John Ott, who has written several books on the subject.

Many people also believe that abnormal levels of melatonin are related to SAD, because melatonin is involved in the body's reaction to light and dark, and affects brain function. Melatonin also helps set the body's internal clock. Some SAD patients have been found to have an unusual delay in their melatonin rhythms. Taking melatonin at night could help, but on the other hand it could make things worse. Melatonin secretion peaks around midnight. It normally increases in winter; in the summer months it drops in women and is unchanged in men.

I don't really know the consequences of taking melatonin on a long-term basis. But for short periods of time it's probably okay. I'd suggest no more than 1 milligram taken at bedtime.

You ask about feverfew (*Tenacetum parthenium*) and serotonin. I don't think the method by which feverfew works for migraine is known. And I don't think we know that feverfew affects serotonin uptake. But feverfew is harmless and would be interesting to try. I'd like to know the results. I'd get an extract of feverfew that is standardized for content of parthenolides. Take one tablet or capsule twice a day over a couple of months and see if you notice an effect.

There is a national support group in the U.K. for people with SAD (see Other Resources p.82 for the address).

Can Zinc Cure
the Common Cold?

Q:

I've heard some talk about zinc lozenges as a cure for the common cold. Is there any validity to this claim? If it's true, where can I find the lozenges?

A:

Zinc gluconate lozenges do have a lot of enthusiasts, although in my experience, reports from users vary. Research on zinc has also delivered mixed results, but one recent study at the Cleveland Clinic found the mineral to cut the duration of a cold in half. No one, however, has found a cure for the common cold.

In the Cleveland study, 50 people with colds sucked on Cold-Eeze lozenges (13 milligrams each) every two hours. Their symptoms cleared up four days sooner than the coughing, runny noses, and sore throats of a comparable group that didn't use the lozenges. Michael Macknin, who designed the research, thinks the zinc ions traveled from the mouth to the nose, where they prevented the viruses that cause colds from settling into the respiratory pathways.

You should be aware that daily doses of zinc above 100 milligrams may depress immunity. And zinc can upset some people's stomachs, so make sure you've eaten before sucking on the lozenges. A lot of people don't like the taste of the lozenges, either.

I personally haven't experienced great benefits from zinc lozenges, but I think they are worth trying. You can buy them in health food stores or regular pharmacies. Some say that the newer zinc acetate lozenges work better than standard forms though these may be difficult to find in the U.K.

Resources

Books by Andrew Weil, M.D.

8 Weeks to Optimum Health: A Proven Program for Taking Full Advantage of Your Body's Natural Healing Power. London: Little, Brown, 1997.

Spontaneous Healing: How to Discover and Enhance Your Body's Natural Ability to Maintain and Heal Itself. London: Little, Brown, 1995.

Natural Health, Natural Medicine: A Comprehensive Manual for Wellness and Self-Care. Rev. ed. London: Little, Brown, 1997.

Health and Healing: Understanding Conventional and Alternative Medicine. Rev. ed. Boston: Houghton Mifflin, 1995.

From Chocolate to Morphine: Everything You Need to Know About Mind-Altering Drugs, with Winifred Rosen. Rev. ed. Boston: Houghton Mifflin, 1993.

The Natural Mind: An Investigation of Drugs and the Higher Consciousness. Rev. ed. Boston: Houghton Mifflin, 1986.

The Marriage of the Sun and the Moon: A Quest for Unity in Consciousness. Boston: Houghton Mifflin, 1980.

Other Recommended Books

Benson, Herbert. *The Relaxation Response.* New York: William Morrow, 1975.

Chester, Laura. *Lupus Novice: Towards Self Healing.* Barrytown, New York: Station Hill Press, 1987.

Keville, Kathi, with Peter Korn. *Herbs for Health and Healing: The Illustrated Encyclopedia of Herbs.* Emmaus, Pennsylvania: Rodale Press, 1996.

Northrup, Christiane, M.D. *Women's Bodies, Women's Wisdom: Creating Physical and Emotional Health and Healing.* New York: Bantam Books, 1995.

Schwartz, Cheryl. *Four Paws, Five Directions.* Berkeley: Celestial Arts, 1996.

Washnis, George J., and Richard Z. Hricak. *Discovery*

of Magnetic Health: A Health Care Alternative.
Rockville, Maryland: Nova Publishing, 1993.

Other Resources

Institute of Complementary Medicine
PO Box 194
London SE1 1QZ
Tel: 0171 237 5165
Holds the Britsh Register of Complementary
Practitioners.

SAD Association
PO Box 989
London SW7 2PZ
Tel: 01903 814942

Program in Integrative Medicine

At the University of Arizona Health Sciences Center,
Tucson, Arizona. For more information, visit the Web
site: http://www.ahsc.arizona.edu/integrative_medi-
cine. Or write: Center for Integrative Medicine, P.O.
Box 64089, Tucson, AZ 85718.

Newsletter

If you would like more information on my lectures

and informational products, including my monthly newsletter, *Self Healing*, please write to: Andrew Weil, M.D., P.O. Box 457, Vail, AZ 85641.

On the Web

'Ask Dr. Weil' answers health questions daily on Time Warner's Pathfinder Network (www.drweil.com).

Index

Acidophilus, 25

Acupuncture, for pets, 1–3

Alcohol
  hangovers, 33–34
  herbal treatments and,
    4–5

Aloe vera, 40, 53

American ginseng (*Panax
    quinquefolius*), 13

Antibiotics, 6, 7

Antihistamines, 35

Arnica, 39–40

Arthritis, 46, 47

Asian ginseng (*Panax
    ginseng*), 13

Bee stings, 6–8

Benson, Herbert, 69

Beta-carotene, 9–11

Bilberry extract, 55–56

Black currant oil, 47, 58

Blue-green algae, 12–13

Breathing, 31–32, 59,
    62–63

Bruises, 39–40

B vitamins, 5, 34, 53

Caffeine, 58

Calcium, 58–59

Cancer
  beta-carotene and, 9–10
  in pets, 1–3

Cephalexin, 6, 7

Chamomile tea, 71

Chester, Laura, 48

Chi (qi), 1–2

Chicken soup, 15–16

Chocolate, 58

Cholesterol, 17–19

Chromium, 20–21

Cigarette smoking,
    quitting, 61–63

Claritin, 35

Coghill, Roger, 49

Colds
  chicken soup and, 15–16
  echinacea and, 7, 26–27
  zinc lozenges and, 78–79
Colloidal minerals, 22–23
Congeners, 34

Dehydration, 33
DGL (deglycyrrhizinated
    licorice), 70, 71
Diet
  cholesterol and, 17
  for lupus, 47
  for premenstrual
      syndrome (PMS), 58
  for smokers, 63
Digestive disorders, 70–72
Dong quai (*Angelica
    sinensis*), 59
Douching, 24-25

Echinacea (*Echinacea
    purpura*), 7, 26–27
Exercise
  cholesterol and, 18
  for premenstrual
      syndrome (PMS), 58
  stress reduction and, 32

Feverfew (*Tanacetum

parthenium), 47,
    76–77
Fleas, 28–30
Forgetting, 31–32
Four Paws, Five Directions
    (Schwartz), 2
Free radicals, 10

Gamma linolenic acid
    (GLA), 47, 58
Garlic, 37–38, 53
Ginger 47
Ginseng, 13, 67
Guided imagery, 47

Hangovers, 33–34
Hay fever, 35–36
HDL (high-density
    lipoprotein)
    cholesterol, 19
Head lice, 43–45
Heartburn, 70, 71
Heart disease, beta-
    carotene and, 10
Herbal treatments
  for alcoholism, 4–5
  for arthritis, 47
  for bruises, 39–40
  dosages, 37–38
  for hay fever, 35-36

Index

Herbal Treatments *cont.*
  for head lice, 44–45
  for insect stings, 6–7
  for low energy, 13
  for nose-bleeding, 55
  for pets, 2
      for premenstrual
      syndrome (PMS),
      59
  for SAD (seasonal
      affective disorder),
      76–77
  for stamina, 67
  for vaginal infections,
      25
Hickey, 39–40
HIV, Kombucha tea for,
      41–42
Hypertension, 69
Hypnotherapy, 47

Immune system, 41–42,
      46–48, 53, 72
Insecticides, 28–29
Insect stings, 6–8
Interferon, 26

Keville, Kathi, 40, 67
Kombucha tea, 41–42
Kudzu (*Pueraria*), 4

LDL (low-density
      lipoprotein)
      cholesterol, 19
Lice, 43–45
Licorice, 67, 70
Low energy, 13
Lung cancer, 9–10
Lupus, 46–48
*Lupus Novice: Towards Self
      Healing* (Chester), 48

Macknin, Michael, 78
Magnesium, 58–59
Magnet therapy, 49–51
Maitake (*Grifola frondosa*)
      mushrooms, 2
Massage, 60
Meditation, 5, 68–69
Melatonin, 76
Memory loss, 31–32
Meridians, 1–2
Milk thistle (*Silybum
      marianum*), 5, 34
Mosquitoes, 52–53

Neutrophils, 15
Niacin, 18–19
Nicotine, 61–62
Northrup, Christiane,
      24–25

Nose-bleeding, 54–56

Ott, John, 76

Pain reduction
  magnet therapy and,
    50
  for pets, 1–3
Peppermint tea, 71
Pets
  acupuncture for, 1–3
  fleas and, 28–30
Placebo, 16
Premenstrual syndrome
    (PMS), 57–59
Pyrethrins, 29

Reishi (Ganoderma
    lucidum) mushrooms,
    2
Relaxation Response, The
    (Benson), 69
Rolfing, 60

SAD (seasonal affective
    disorder), 75–77
Schizandra, 67
Schwartz, Cheryl, 2
Serotonin, 76, 77
Silver products, 23

Skin-So-Soft, 52
Smoking, quitting, 61–63
Snoring, 64–65
Stamina, 67
Steroid drugs, 35–36
Stinging nettle (Urtica
    dioica), 36
Stitches, 66–67
Stress reduction, 31–32
Surgery, healing after, 14

T cells, 26, 42
Tea tree oil (Melaleuca
    alternifolia), 7, 25
Tiger Balm, 53
Tobacco, 61–63
Transcendental meditation
    (TM), 68–69
Turmeric, 47

Urine therapy, 73–74

Vaginal infections, 25
Vitamin A, 11
Vitamin B-3 (niacin),
    18–19
Vitamin C, 14, 55
Vitamin E, 55
Vitex (Vitex agnus-castus),
    59

Women's Antioxidant and
    Cardiovascular Study,
    11
*Women's Bodies, Women's
    Wisdom* (Northrup),
    24–25

Yarrow (*Achillea
    millefolium*), 55
Yoga, 5

Zinc lozenges, colds and,
    78-79

Acknowledgments

Richard Pine, Judith Curr, Elisa Wares, and Scott Fagan